Vegan Diet:

A Complete Guide for Beginners: Quick and Easy Vegan Recipes for Weight Loss and a Healthy Lifestyle

Sarah Maddington

© 2018

© Copyright 2017 - All rights reserved.

The contents of this book may not be reproduced, duplicated or transmitted without direct written permission from the author.

Under no circumstances will any legal responsibility or blame be held against the publisher for any reparation, damages, or monetary loss due to the information herein, either directly or indirectly.

<u>Legal Notice:</u>

This book is copyright protected. This is only for personal use. You cannot amend, distribute, sell, use, quote or paraphrase any part or the content within this book without the consent of the author.

<u>Disclaimer Notice:</u>

Please note the information contained within this document is for educational and entertainment purposes only. Every attempt has been made to provide accurate, up to date and reliable complete information. No warranties of any kind are expressed or implied. Readers acknowledge that the author is not engaging in the rendering of legal, financial, medical or professional advice. The content of this book has been derived from various sources. Please consult a licensed professional before attempting any techniques outlined in this book.

By reading this document, the reader agrees that under no circumstances are is the author responsible for any losses, direct or indirect, which are incurred as a result of the use of information contained within this document, including, but not limited to, —errors, omissions, or inaccuracies

About Sarah Maddington

Sarah Maddington was born and raised in Manchester, UK. She is a Weight-Loss coach, Dietitian, Professional Chef and a mother of two. After finishing high school, she moved to London to pursue her dreams to study culinary.

In the past, Sarah was very overweight and suffered many health problems. She struggled with weight issues and found it difficult to maintain the balance between her career and her health.

It wasn't until after giving birth to her eldest daughter Sally, did she realise that she had to take her health more seriously if she wanted to become a role model for her children.
She lost 57 pounds in 6 months. Today, she wants to inspire beautiful people around the world to take control of the health so they can get back the life they deserve.

Table of Contents

Introduction

Our society has seen a lot of change in recent years. The way we do business, science and technology, communication, travel and so on. But there's one thing hasn't seen much change in the last few decades, our diet. With all the junk going around, fast food, doctors giving mixed advice, how do we know what's actually good for us?

There are many different types of diets going around, from the prehistoric paleo diet, to a more modern ketogenic diet, and of course the typical vegetarian diet. One diet, the vegan diet, has slowly gained popularity over the years, equating to nearly 1% in the USA alone. This may not seem like much, but given our animalistic nature to want to eat meat, it might seem quite absurd to many that people wouldn't want to eat meat at all, let alone any animal bi-products such as milk, cheese, eggs and even arguably honey.

The vegan diet or veganism is a diet which does not consist of any meat or animal products, including dairy products. Alternatively, one way of looking at veganism is a diet that excludes any exploitation of any animals.

Although honey is a contentious topic in the vegan community, some vegans choose to eat honey due to the health benefits. However, for the sake of diversity, recipes in this book will include honey. Though it's not necessary to use honey within the recipes.

Advantages Vegan Diet

Economic costs

There are many health benefits to going vegan as well as it being a more economical way of life. There is a huge misconception that going vegan is more expensive but you'll find that going vegan can actually save you money by buying fresh fruits and vegetables that are in season. One of the most expensive ingredients for the modern meal is meat, but when you cut that out your grocery bill can actually go down.

Health benefits

There are many proven health benefits when it comes to becoming a vegan. The vegan diet can help defend against osteoporosis, it promotes weight loss by lowering the total fat that you're ingesting, helps with high blood pressure, reduces cholesterol and can even help prevent diabetes.

In this book you'll find a large number of vegan diet recipes that are good for any time of the day, so you never have to worry about breaking your diet due to convenience. Most of the recipes listed can be taken on the go too!

Simple and easy

Although to some people veganism may sound boring and flavourless, it revolves around little to no cooking. Most vegans tend to eat mainly raw food, primarily due to the belief that frying food destroys the living bacteria within food. Because of this, vegans tend to follow a path of raw, mixed or cooked foods. The benefits of the vegan diet lies within its simplicity. It is much simpler to eat some fruits on the go, eat some raw carrots, nuts and other vegetables instead of actually cooking them, thus saving more time and stress of what to eat.

Environmental Costs

It is obvious that one of the biggest benefits when it comes to the vegan diet is the level of environmental cost. Not only is meat the largest producer of greenhouse gases, the vegan diet has very little negative impact on the environment. Growing fruits and vegetables is a very sustainable practice, and in a world where we have less land and more people to feed, this could be a great solution.

Disadvantages of the Vegan Diet

Acceptance

The biggest issue faced with veganism is the lack of acceptance of the diet. Unlike it's sibling the vegetarian diet, many vegans find in restaurants there is a lack of vegan-based meals on the menu (until this book). There is a growing demand for vegan-based restaurants, however, the vegan diet is still in early stages of adoption.

Uncomfortable

It is true that making the transition from a meat-based diet to a vegan-based diet is uncomfortable. Eating something you don't like, feeling a way you don't want to feel. Which is why in the following chapter, we will go through different ways we can tackle the issue. It involves rewiring your brain and breaking old eating patterns, however, if you really want to change anything is possible. Overtime your body will adjust to the change, but the initial process will be uncomfortable.

Lack of protein?

The vegan diet is known to get a lot of scrutiny, where critics claim the vegan diet is not a balanced diet for the average person. There is a misconception that vegans don't get enough protein in their diet, due to non-existent meat intake, however, this is far from the truth. If we look deeper into proteins, there are many forms of proteins, in fact the body breaks down proteins into what is known as amino acids, which is what is actually used to sustain muscle and develop muscles. These proteins can be found in various forms, primarily as we know, from meat, such as chicken and beef. However, there are also plant proteins. In fact, as crazy as it might sound, plants actually contain more protein per gram than meat does. If we eat 100 grams of plants, it's significantly more protein than 100 grams of beef.

Additionally, if we look at high protein based foods such as peanuts, almonds, and other nuts, as well as, our soy based products, lack of protein is really not an issue faced with the vegan-based diet.

How to begin

For some people, it can be easier to transition in steps instead of all at once. It is understandable that if you eat meat your whole life, going cold turkey into a fruit and vegetable-based diet can be overwhelming, or underwhelming (for the stomach). My recommendation is to start slowly. Some individuals are uncomfortable with the idea of eating just fruit and vegetables as meal, and that's fine, if so, start by incorporating more vegetables into your day. If you're used to only eating meat and dislike your veggies, the only way forward is to actually eat them. You'll find that your taste buds and appetite will change over time and adjust accordingly. You'll feel less hungry and crave less sugar and greasy foods in the long term.

If you're coming from a heavy meat and dairy-based diet, start by eating one vegan-based meal a day. Try that for 1-2 weeks, and if you feel that you can handle more, start increase the meals per day. If you start counting, you'll notice you're making progress. If you feel that one meal is too much for you to start off, you can start off with adding extra vegetables and fruit on top of your current diet, and slowly reduce meat and dairy intake.

In this book we have created delicious recipes so you can begin your journey to become a vegan. Quick and easy tips so you can cook in the comfort of your home. Let's begin!

Breakfast Recipes

Breakfast is the most important meal of the day, but usually people think of eggs and bacon the moment they hear the word. Those people don't know what they're missing without these delicious vegan breakfast recipes as a part of their morning routine.

Green Breakfast Sandwich

Serves: 1

Ingredients:

Patty:

- Vegan Sausage Patty
- Dash Chipotle Powder
- Sea Salt & Black Pepper to taste
- Vegetable Oil

Kale Sauté:

- 2 Cups Kale, Torn
- 1 Teaspoon Olive Oil
- 2 Tablespoons Pumpkin Seeds
- Sea Salt & Pepper to Taste
- ½ Shallot, Sliced Thin

Jalapeno Mayo:

- 1 ½ Tablespoons Vegan Mayonnaise

- ½ Teaspoon Chipotle Powder
- ½ Teaspoon Jalapeno, Dried
- 1 Tablespoon Lime Juice, for Thinning
- 2 Slices Avocado, Rubbed in Lemon Juice
- 1 English Muffin, Toasted

Directions:

1. Add a drizzle of your oil to your pan, turning the heat to high. Place your shallots in the pan, cooking for about a minute. Your shallots should start to brown, and then place them in a small bowl.
2. Place your heat on high, and then place in your sausage patty. Add your spices to your patty, and then drizzle more oil into your pan if necessary. Cook for one to two minutes per side. The edges should begin to brown, and then set your patty aside.
3. Add your kale sauté ingredients to the pan while it's still warm. Cover, and then let it steam for a minute. The kale should become wilted, and then you can turn off the heat. Toss this into you shallots, and then mix together. Add in your pumpkin seeds, mixing again.
4. Mix everything for your jalapeno vegan mayonnaise together, and then assemble to eat.

Buckwheat & Apple Pancakes

Serves: 2

Ingredients:

Dry Ingredients:

- 2 Teaspoon Baking Powder
- 1 ¾ Cups Buckwheat Flour
- 2 Tablespoons Coconut Sugar
- ¼ Teaspoon Sea Salt, Fine
- 2 Teaspoons Cinnamon
- ¼ Teaspoon Vanilla Powder

Wet Ingredients:

- 1 Flax Egg
- 1 ¼ Cup + 2 Tablespoons Almond Milk
- 2 Tablespoons Coconut Oil, Melted
- 1 Cup Apple, Peeled & Chopped Fine

Caramel & Coconut Apples

- 1 Teaspoon Coconut Oil
- 1 Teaspoon Cinnamon
- 2 Tablespoons Coconut Sugar
- ¼ Teaspoon Water
- 1 Gala Apple, Peeled & Sliced

Directions:

1. Start by preparing your flax egg. You need to mix a tablespoon of ground flax seed with three tablespoons of water, and then let it rest for five full minutes.

2. Sift and whisk all of your dry ingredients together in a bowl.

3. Mix your almond milk and flax egg together before adding it to your dry ingredients.

4. Let your pancake batter rest for fifteen minutes, and then add an additional two tablespoons almond milk, chopped apple and coconut oil.

5. Place your coconut oil in your frying pan, and then turn the heat to low.

6. Pour in a ¼ cup of batter into your pan, and then cook for two to three minutes on each side. Repeat until all of your batter is used.

7. Take another pan, and melt your coconut oil for your caramel apples in it, and then add in your cinnamon, water and sugar. Make sure to mix well.

8. Serve your apples over your pancakes.

Gingerbread Waffles

Serves: 2

Ingredients:

Dry Ingredients:

- 1 Tablespoon Flax seeds, Ground
- ¼ Teaspoon Baking Soda
- 1 Cup Spelt Flour
- 2 Teaspoons Baking Powder
- ¼ Teaspoon Sea Salt, Fine
- 1 ½ Teaspoons Cinnamon
- 2 Teaspoons Ginger
- 4 Tablespoons Coconut Sugar

Wet Ingredients:

- 2 Tablespoons Black Strap Molasses
- 1 ½ Tablespoons Coconut Oil
- 1 Tablespoon Apple Cider Vinegar
- 1 Cup Almond Milk

Directions:

1. Start by greasing and preheating your waffle iron. It's best to set it on four. If you don't have a waffle iron, you can use this recipe to make pancakes instead.
2. Place all dry ingredients in a bowl, mixing together.
3. Mix all wet ingredients in a separate bowl, stirring well.
4. Mix your wet and dry ingredients together until combined, but make sure not to overmix. It's okay to have a few lumps.

5. Pour part of your mixture into your waffle iron and cook. Repeat this until you make all six waffles.

6. Serve immediately while warm.

Grits & Avocado Bowl

Serves: 4

Ingredients:

- 1 Block Tofu, Extra Firm & Sliced into Strips
- ¼ Cup Soy Sauce, Low Sodium
- ½ Teaspoon Onion Powder
- 1 Teaspoon Turmeric
- 1 Tablespoon Olive Oil
- ½ Teaspoon Onion Powder
- 4 Serving Grits + Enough Water to Make
- ½ Cup Nutritional Yeast
- 2 Tablespoons Coconut Oil
- 1 Avocado, Sliced
- Sea Salt & Pepper to Taste

Directions:

1. Start by heating your oven to 425.
2. Start by whisking your soy sauce, onion powder, olive oil and turmeric together in order to make your marinade. Toss in your tofu strips, letting them sit for fifteen minutes.
3. Place them on a baking sheet, baking for fifteen minutes. Slip the strips, baking for another fifteen minutes.
4. Prepare your grits as per your package instructions.
5. Stir your nutritional yeast and coconut oil into your grits.
6. Divide into four servings, topping with tofu strips, avocado, and seasoning with salt and pepper.

Asparagus & Tomato Quiche

Serves: 8

Ingredients:

Crust:

- 1 ½ Cups All Purpose Flour
- ½ Cup Almond Butter
- ½ Teaspoon Sea Salt, Fine
- 3 Tablespoons Water, Ice Cold

Filling:

- ¼ Cup White Onion, Minced
- 1 Tablespoon Vegetable Oil
- 1 Cup Asparagus, Fresh & Chopped
- 3 Tablespoons Tomatoes, Dried & Chopped
- 14 Ounces Tofu, Firm & Drained
- 3 Tablespoons Nutritional Yeast
- 1 Tablespoon All Purpose Flour
- 1 Tablespoon Almond Milk
- 1 Teaspoon Minced Onion, Dehydrated
- 2 Teaspoon Lemon Juice, Fresh
- 1 Teaspoon Spicy Mustard
- ½ Teaspoon Sea Salt, Fine
- ½ Teaspoon Turmeric
- ½ Teaspoon Liquid Smoke
- 3 Tablespoons Basil, Fresh & Chopped
- 1/3 Cup Vegan Cheese of Your Choice

- Sea Salt & Black Pepper to Taste

Directions:

1. Get out a nine inch pan and then spray it before setting it to the side. Turn your oven to 350.

2. Combine your flour and salt in a bowl to make your crust, and then add your almond butter in small chunks. Cut the dough to resemble pea sized pieces, and then add your cold water. Turnover, using a floured surface, bringing it together.

3. Press your crust into your pie pan, baking for ten minutes.

4. Remove it from the oven, and let it cool while you start to make your filling.

5. Heat a tablespoon of oil over medium heat, adding in your onions. Sauté until they become translucent, which will take about three minutes. Add in your tomatoes and asparagus, sautéing for another three minutes. The asparagus should become slightly tender. Remove it from heat before setting it aside.

6. Take your tofu and place it in your food processor. Add in your almond milk, nutritional yeast, turmeric, flour, onions, liquid smoke, and sea salt and lemon juice. Pulse until smooth. Transfer to a bowl before adding in your basil, asparagus mixture, and vegan cheese. Stir everything together, seasoning with salt and pepper.

7. Spoon the filling onto you're curst, smoothing the top out. Bake for thirty to forty-five minutes. The top should be

browned, and a knife inserted into the center should come out clean.

8. Allow it to cool for twenty minutes before slicing, and then serve warm.

Fig & Oatmeal Bake Topped to Perfection

Serves: 6

Ingredients:

Oatmeal Bake:

- 1 ½ Teaspoons Baking Powder
- ½ Cup Cashews
- 1 Cup Figs, Dried & Quartered
- 2 Cups Rolled Oats
- ¼ Teaspoon Sea Salt, Fine
- ½ Teaspoon Cinnamon
- 2 Cups Almond Milk
- ½ Cup Fig Spread
- 1 Teaspoon Vanilla Extract, Pure

Streusel Topping:

- ¾ Cup Coconut Sugar
- ¼ Cup Vegan Buttery Spread
- 1 Teaspoon Cinnamon
- 1 Tablespoon Water
- ¾ Cup Flour

Caramelized Pears:

- 2 Bosc Pears, Sliced Thin
- ¼ Teaspoon Cinnamon
- 1 Teaspoon Coconut Oil

Directions:

1. Start by turning your oven to 375.

2. Combine your dried figs, cashews, baking powder, oats, cinnamon and salt together.

3. In another bowl whisk your almond milk, fig spread and vanilla extract together. Make sure it's mixed well.

4. Mix your dry and wet ingredients together, mixing well.

5. Grease a nine by nine pan, and then pour the mixture in. bake for twenty minutes.

6. Combine all ingredients for your streusel topping, making sure to combine well.

7. Top your oats with streusel after baking, and then place in the oven for another ten to fifteen minutes, baking your topping on.

8. Heat a skillet using medium-high heat, and then add in your coconut oil for your pears. Add your pears to the skillet when it's hot, sprinkling cinnamon over them. Cook each side for two to three minutes.

9. Allow your fig oatmeal to cook for ten minutes before topping with pears and serving.

Vegan French Toast

Serves: 4

Ingredients:

- 1 Banana, Large
- ½ Teaspoon Cinnamon
- 1 Teaspoon Vanilla Extract, Pure
- 1 Tablespoon Maple Syrup, Pure
- ¾ Cup Coconut Milk, Full Fat
- 1 Tablespoon Vegan Butter
- 4-6 Slices Bread, Day Old

Directions:

1. Take a food processor, blending your coconut milk, vanilla extract, maple syrup, cinnamon and banana together. Blend until it has a smoothie consistency.
2. Pour this mixture into a shallow bowl that will fit your bread slices.
3. Heat your vegan butter in a frying pan over medium heat, and then dip your bread into your batter. Make sure both sides are coated, and then fry for one to two minutes per side. It should turn a golden brown.
4. Serve warm.

Tempeh Sweet Potato Scramble

Serves: 4

Ingredients:

- 2 Tablespoons Olive Oil
- 1 Small Onion, Diced
- 1 Small Sweet Potato, Finely Diced
- 2 Cloves Garlic, Minced
- 8 Ounces Tempeh, Crumbled
- 1 Small Red Bell Pepper, Diced
- 1 Tablespoon Ground Cumin
- 1 Tablespoon Soy Sauce
- 1 Tablespoon Smoked Paprika
- 1 Tablespoon Maple Syrup, Pure
- ½ Lemon, Juiced

For Serving:

- 1 Avocado, Sliced
- 4 Tortillas
- Hot Sauce to Taste
- 2 Scallions, Chopped

Directions:

1. Place your olive oil in a large skillet, turning your heat to medium. Add in your sweet potato, cooking until lightly browned. It should take about five minutes.

2. Add your onion, continuing to sauté until softened. This will take another five minutes, and then add in your garlic, cooking for another minute. Add your tempeh, cooking until browned. This will take another five minutes. You'll need to break some of your tempeh with a spatula.

3. Add your cumin, paprika, soy sauce, pepper, lemon juice and maple syrup. Sauté for another two minutes.

4. Serve on tortillas topped with scallions, hot sauce, and avocado while still warm.

Strawberry & Quinoa Bowl

Serves: 1

Ingredients:

- 1 Cup Quinoa, Cooked
- 1 Tablespoon Liquid Sweetener
- 1 Cup Strawberries, Frozen
- ¾ Cup Water
- ¼ Cup Cashews

Toppings:

- Fresh Blueberries
- Almonds, Sliced

Directions:

1. Add your water, strawberries, liquid sweetener and cashews to a blender. Blend until smooth. It should have a creamy texture.
2. Place your quinoa in a bowl, pouring the mixture over it.
3. Sprinkle with blueberries and almonds before serving.

Tofu Scramble

Serves: 4

Ingredients:

- 1 Small Onion, Chopped
- 2 Tablespoons Vegetable Oil
- 28 Ounces Tofu, ETrac Firm
- 1 Small Red Bell Pepper, Chopped Fine
- 1 Small Green Bell Pepper, Chopped Fine
- ½ Teaspoon Ground Cumin
- ½ Teaspoon Ground Coriander
- 1 ½ Teaspoons Ground Turmeric
- 15 Ounces Black Beans, Canned, Rinsed & Drained
- ¼ Cup Cilantro, Chopped Coarse
- Sea Salt & Black Pepper to Taste
- 4-6 Whole Wheat Tortillas, Warmed

Directions:

1. Place your tofu on a plate, lined with paper towels. This will allow the liquid to be absorbed. Mash your tofu with a fork.
2. Heat your oil in a skillet using medium-high heat. Add in your peppers and onions, cooking while stirring often. This should take three to four minutes, and they should soften slightly.
3. Stir your coriander and cumin in, cooking for about a minute so that they become fragrant.
4. Add in your tofu and turmeric.

5. Add your beans, cooking while stirring often for one to two minutes.

6. Add in your cilantro, seasoning with salt and pepper.

7. Serve in tortillas while still warm.

31

Tapioca Porridge

Serves: 4

Ingredients:

- 1/3 Cup White Sugar
- ½ Cup Coconut Flakes, Unsweetened & Toasted
- 1 ½ Teaspoons Lemon Juice, Fresh
- 13.5 Ounces Coconut Milk, Light
- ¼ Cup Tapioca, Small Pearl

Directions:

1. Place two cups of water and your tapioca in a saucepan with a heavy bottom. Allow it to soak in the water for a half hour before adding in your sugar and coconut milk.
2. Stir and bring it to a boil using medium heat, making sure to stir constantly.
3. Reduce the heat, allowing it to simmer for fifteen minutes. The tapioca should become translucent, and you'll want to stir frequently so it doesn't scorch.
4. Add in your lemon juice, taking it off heat and garnishing with coconut flakes before serving.

Banana Nut & Hot Chocolate Oatmeal

Serves: 4

Ingredients:

- 2 Cups old Fashioned Rolled Oats
- 2 Cups Almond Milk
- 2 Large Bananas, Ripened & Diced
- ¼ Teaspoon Almond Extract, Pure
- ¼ Teaspoon Vanilla Extract, Pure
- Sea Salt to Taste
- 2 Tablespoons Cocoa Powder, Unsweetened
- 2 Tablespoons Honey, Raw
- 1/3 Cup Walnuts, Toasted & Chopped
- ¼ Teaspoon Cinnamon
- 2 Tablespoons Chocolate Chips, Semi-Sweet

Directions:

1. Bring your almond milk to a boil, mixing in 1 ¾ cup water, almond extract, vanilla extract, diced bananas and sea salt to a boil using high heat. It's best to use a large saucepan.

2. Add in your oats, cocoa powder, and a tablespoon of honey before reducing your heat to medium.

3. Cook while stirring frequently. Your oats should be cooked fully, which will take six to seven minutes.

4. Divide between four bowls, topping with walnuts, a tablespoon of honey, cinnamon, sliced bananas and chocolate chips.

Vegan Banana Bread

Serves: 16

Ingredients:

- 1 Cup White Sugar
- 1 ½ Cups Bananas, Ripe & Mashed
- ½ Cup Coconut Oil, Refined & Melted
- 1 Teaspoon Vanilla Extract, Pure
- ½ Cup Walnuts, Chopped
- ½ Teaspoon Sea Salt, Fine
- ¾ Teaspoon Baking Soda
- 2 Cups All Purpose Flour
- 1 Teaspoon Apple Cider Vinegar
- ¼ Cup Almond Milk, Vanilla & Unsweetened

Directions:

1. Start by heating your oven to 350, and then grease a 9x5x3 inch loaf pan.
2. Beat your bananas, coconut oil, sugar and vanilla until smooth in a large bowl. Add in your almond milk, and then stir in your vinegar.
3. Add in your baking soda, and then stir in your slat. Stir until everything is just moistened.
4. Add in your walnuts before pouring the mixture into your pan.
5. Bake for an hour to one hour and ten minutes. A toothpick inserted into the middle should come out clean. Allow it to cool for ten minutes before loosening the

sides, and removing from the pan. Allow it to cool for an hour on a cooling rack before slicing.

Scallion Pancakes

Serves: 4

Ingredients:

Dough:

- 2 Tablespoons Water, Lukewarm
- ¾ Cup Water, Lukewarm
- 2 Teaspoons Canola Oil
- 2 Cups All Purpose Flour
- 1 Teaspoon Sea Salt, Fine
- ½ Cup Vegan Yogurt, Plain

Scallions:

- ½ Teaspoon Sea Salt, Fine
- ½ Teaspoon Lime Juice, Fresh
- 2 Cups Green Onions, Chopped Fine
- ½ Teaspoon Black Pepper

Directions:

1. In a bowl mix your flour, sea salt, yogurt, and canola oil.
2. Slowly mix in ¾ cups lukewarm water while mixing, and then add the remaining two tablespoons.
3. Rolle the dough into the bowl, and it should become sticky.
4. Cover, and let it sit for thirty minutes.
5. In another bowl, add your scallions, sea salt, black pepper and lime juice, mixing well before placing it to the side.

6. Heat a griddle over medium heat, and make a small ball out of the dough.

7. Flatten it, rolling it into a small circle.

8. Add a tablespoon of scallions, and then fold the edges over.

9. Press it down, and then turn it over before rolling it in a circle again. Remember that it doesn't have to be perfect.

10. Spray your griddle before placing the pancake in it. Cook each side for two minutes until it browns evenly.

11. Set it aside, and repeat the process until all of your dough is used up.

Pumpkin Muffins

Serves: 12

Ingredients:

- 1 Apple, Chopped
- 1 Cup Pumpkin Puree
- 1 Teaspoon Baking Powder
- 1 Teaspoon Baking Soda
- 2 Tablespoons Pumpkin Pie Spice
- ¾ Cup Coconut Palm Sugar
- 2 Cups Almond Flour
- 1 Cup Oats
- ¼ Cup Coconut Oil, Melted
- ½ Teaspoon Almond Extract, Pure
- ½ Teaspoon Vanilla Extract, Pure
- 6 Tablespoons Water
- 2 Tablespoons Flax Seeds, Ground

Directions:

1. Start by heating your oven to 350.
2. Mix your sugar, oats, pumpkin pie spice, almond flour, baking powder and baking powder together in a large bowl.
3. In another bowl, mix your flax seeds and water, to create the flax egg equivalent of two eggs. Allow it to thicken by setting it aside for a few minutes.
4. In another bowl mix your coconut oil, apple, pumpkin puree, extracts, and flax eggs together, making sure to

combine well. Fold your wet ingredients into your dry ingredients.

5. Spray a muffin tin using a coconut oil spray, and then evenly distribute your batter. Bake for twenty-three to twenty-five minutes. It should be lightly browned, and a toothpick once inserted into the middle should come out clean.

6. Allow your muffins to cool before serving.

Omelet Muffins

Serves: 6

Ingredients:

- 1 Cup Chickpea Flour
- 3 Tablespoons Nutritional Yeast
- 1 ½ Tablespoons Apple Cider Vinegar
- 1 Teaspoon Mustard
- 2 Tablespoons Olive Oil
- ¾ Cup Water
- ½ Cup Coconut Milk, Lite
- ¼ Teaspoon Black Pepper
- ¼ Teaspoon Sea Salt, Fine
- /2 Teaspoon Garlic Powder
- ½ Teaspoon Onion Powder
- ¼ Teaspoon Baking Powder
- ½ Teaspoon Turmeric
- 1 Shallot, Minced
- ½ Red Bell Pepper, Diced
- 1 Carrot, Diced
- 1 Cup Kale, Chopped
- 2 Tablespoons Olives, Diced
- 1 Tablespoon Olive Oil

Directions:

1. Heat a tablespoon of olive oil, in a skillet, and then add your bell pepper, carrots and shallots. Sauté until slightly softened, which will take two to three minutes.

2. Add in your kale and olives, sautéing until the kale has wilted slightly. This should take one to two minutes, and then remove from heat before setting it aside.

3. Preheat your oven to 450, and then grease a muffin tin before setting it to the side.

4. Combine your chickpea flour, water, and coconut milk before whisking it together. Add all remaining ingredients to the mix, making sure it's well combined.

5. Divide your sautéed vegetables evenly between the muffin tins before pouring the muffin mixture over it. Fill it almost to the top. You should get six to eight muffins.

6. Use a fork to stir the vegetables and batter together, and then bake for fifteen minutes. Lower the temperature to 430, baking for another ten to fifteen minutes. Remember that a toothpick should be able to be inserted to the center and then come out clean.

7. Allow it to cool for a few minutes before serving.

Peanut & Date Congee

Serves: 2

Ingredients:

- 1/8 Cup Peanuts, Raw
- ¼ Cup Jasmine White Rice
- 4 Slices Ginger
- 3 Cups Water
- 4 Dates, Dried
- Sea Salt & Pepper to Taste

Directions:

1. Soak your rice and peanuts in water, but do so separately. You'll want to soak them overnight. Soak the dates overnight as well.
2. Drain the soaking water away from all of your ingredients, and then crush the rice with your hands.
3. Bring two cups of water to a boil before adding your dates, ginger, rice and peanuts together.
4. Allow it to continue to boil, but stir to prevent sticking or burning.
5. The lid should be half open so that the water doesn't overflow. You need to let it boil until the rice disintegrates. When it starts sputtering, add a ½ cup of water.
6. Add another ½ cup water once it starts to sputter again. you should now have three cups of water.

7. Leave it on the stove, allowing it to reach the desired consistency. This should take about forty-five minutes.

8. Add salt and pepper when done before serving.

Quinoa & Vegetable Flakes

Serves: 1

Ingredients:

- ¼ Teaspoon Smoked Paprika
- 1/8 Teaspoon Cumin
- ¼ Teaspoon Onion Powder
- ¼ Teaspoon Turmeric
- 1 Tablespoon Hemp Seeds
- 1 Tablespoon Nutritional Yeast
- 1/3 Cup Quinoa Flakes
- ¼ Cup Zucchini, Shredded
- Handful Baby Spinach, Torn
- 2/3 Cup + 2 Tablespoons Water

Directions:

1. Combine all of your dry ingredients in a microwave safe bowl before mixing in the spinach, water and zucchini. Make sure everything is mixed well.
2. Microwave on high for ninety seconds to two minutes.
3. Remove carefully, and allow to cool before enjoying.

Mediterranean Oatmeal

Serves: 4

Ingredients:

- 1 Cu Cherry Tomatoes, Sliced
- 1 Cup Spinach, Chopped Coarsely
- ½ Teaspoon Sea Salt
- ¾ Cup Steel Cut Oats
- 2 Cups water
- ¾ Cup Kalamata Olives, Pitted & Chopped Coarsely
- 1 teaspoon Vegan Butter
- ¼ Cup Basil Leaves, Fresh & Chopped Coarsely

Directions:

1. Bring your water to a boil in a saucepan, adding in your oats and salt. Reduce your heat to let it simmer, stirring occasionally until it reaches a risotto texture. This should take about five minutes.
2. Add in your spinach, stirring well until wilted. This will take about two minutes.
3. Add in your olives and tomatoes, and then cook until it's warmed all the way through, which should take two to three minutes.
4. Add in your vegan butter, stirring until melted.
5. Add half of your basil, stirring to combine.
6. Remove from heat, serving while warm. Garnish with black pepper and the remaining basil.

Kale & Tofu Breakfast Bowl

Serves: 1

Ingredients:

- 6 Ounces Tofu, Extra Firm
- 1 Tablespoon Coconut Oil
- 1 Tablespoon Nutritional Yeast
- Sea Salt & Black Pepper to Taste
- 3-4 Kale Leaves, Chopped
- ¼ Cup Cabbage, Quick Pickled
- Red Pepper Flakes for Topping
- 1 Dollop Cashew Crème for Topping

Directions:

1. Start by heating a skillet using medium-high heat, and then melt your coconut oil in it.
2. Cut your tofu into three quarter inch cubes, sprinkling them with salt.
3. Add your tofu's to the pan once your oil is hot, and it should sizzle when placed in the pan. Sauté for seven minutes, stirring occasionally. Your tofu should be crispy on all sides, and then add in your nutritional yeast, tossing to coat.
4. Add your kale before lowering the heat. Add in one to two tablespoons of water, helping the kale to cook down. Stir occasionally, cooking until the kale becomes wilted.
5. Transfer to a bowl, topping with your pickled cabbage, red pepper flakes and cashew crème.

Lunch Recipes

Lunch is another important meal of the day, and eating vegan for lunch doesn't have to be hard. These vegan meals are simple to make, and most can be taken on the go too!

Sabich Sandwich

Serves: 3

Ingredients:

- Pita Bread Pockets
- 2 Potatoes, Firm, Peeled & Boiled
- 1 Young Eggplant
- ½ Cup White Beans, Canned, Drained & Rinsed Well
- 1 Tablespoon Vegan Mayonnaise
- ¼ Teaspoon Harissa Paste
- 3 Dill Pickles, Whole
- ½ Cup Humus
- ½ Cup Tabbouleh Salad
- 1/3 Cup Tahini Sauce
- Sea Salt to Taste
- Olive Oil to Taste

Directions:

1. Chop your eggplant into cubes, and then heat up a frying pan with olive oil.

2. Season your eggplant using salt, and then cook your eggplant until it holds it shape but is slightly creamy.

3. Remove from heat, and set them aside.

4. Slice your boiled potato into thin slices. Combine your white beans, mayonnaise and harissa paste together in another bowl.

5. Slice your dill pickles in vertical slices, and then lay your pitas out.

6. Build your sandwich, and then add hummus onto each pita.

7. Cover half of it with sliced potatoes, and then lay sliced pickle over your potato.

8. Spoon two tablespoons of your white bean mixture on top of your pickles.

9. Add 2-3 tablespoons of cooked eggplant to each sandwich, and then drizzle with tahini sauce.

10. Serve and enjoy!

Asian Noodle Salad

Serves: 3

Ingredients:

- 6.2 Ounces Soba Noodles
- 1 ½ Cups carrot, Grated
- ½ Cup Cilantro, Chopped
- Sesame Seeds to Taste
- 2/3 Cup Cucumber, Sliced Thin
- 2 Cups Red Cabbage, Shredded Thin

Peanut Sauce:

- 1 Lime, Juiced
- ½ Tablespoon Ginger, Grated
- ½ Teaspoon Coconut Sugar
- 2-4 Tablespoons Water
- 2 Cloves Garlic, Minced
- 1 Tablespoon Tamari
- ½ Cup Peanut Butter, Natural

Directions:

1. Start by rinsing and prepping all of your vegetables.
2. In a small bowl, combine all of your peanut sauce ingredients together. Add the amount of water needed to reach your desired consistency.
3. Ring a pot of water to boil, and then cook your noodles per package instructions. Drain, rinsing them with cold water.

4. Add in your carrot, cucumber, cilantro, and cabbage into a bowl. Add in your peanut sauce, mixing well. Gently fold in your noodles.

5. Garnish with sesame seeds before serving immediately.

Vegan Philly Cheesesteak

Serves: 2

Ingredients:

- 7 Ounces Vegan Provolone Slices
- ¼ Teaspoon Onion Powder
- 1 Teaspoon Celery Flakes
- ¼ Teaspoon Garlic Powder
- 8 Ounces Seitan
- ½ Yellow Onion, Sliced
- 1 Green Pepper, Seeded & Sliced
- 4 Tablespoons Olive Oil
- Sea Salt & Black Pepper to Taste
- 2 Vegan French Rolls, Cut in Half

Directions:

1. Start by heating your oven to 375.
2. Heat up your olive oil over medium heat in a large pan. Sauté your onion, seitan, and green pepper together for five minutes. Your seitan should be heated all the way through, and then add your onion powder, garlic powder, salt, pepper and celery flakes.
3. Transfer it to an oven safe pan, and then top with your vegan provolone. Bake for ten minutes. Your "cheese" should have melted.
4. Melt the remaining olive oil in a pan over medium heat, and then toast your French rolls until crispy.

5. Fill your French rolls with your seitan, vegan cheese, onion and green pepper before serving warm.

Creamy Avocado Pasta

Serves: 2

Ingredients:

- 2 Avocados, Pitted & Diced
- 1 Clove Garlic, Minced
- ¼ Cup Water
- ¼ Cup Soy Milk, Unsweetened
- Red Pepper Flakes to Taste
- 2 Cups Pasta, Cooked
- 4 Cherry Tomatoes, Halved for Garnish
- ½ Lemon, Juiced
- Sea Salt to Taste

Directions:

1. Combine your lemon juice, garlic and avocados in a food processor. Blend, and then add in your water and soy milk.
2. Add your red pepper flakes and salt to taste.
3. Serve over your cooked pasta.

Vegan Pesto Pasta

Serves: 4

Ingredients:

- ¼ Cup Olive Oil
- ¼ Cup Water, Hot
- ½ Cup Pine Nuts
- 2 Cups Basil Leaves, Fresh & Packed
- 2 Garlic Cloves, Minced
- 1 lb Pasta
- Sea Salt to Taste

Directions:

1. Cook your pasta like you normally would.
2. Combine your pine nuts, basil and garlic in a blender, blending on low. Slowly add in your olive oil while your blender is running. Add in your h to water next. Add your sea salt, and then continue to blend until you get a smooth and creamy pasta sauce.
3. Drain your pasta, and then toss in your pesto sauce to serve.

Vegan Miso Soup

Serves: 3

Ingredients:

- 4 Cups Water
- 3 Tablespoons Miso
- 1.5 Ounces Noodles
- ½ Cup Onion
- 3.5 Ounces Soft Tofu
- 1 Tablespoon Wakame Seaweed, Dried

Directions:

1. Cook your noodles like you normally would before draining them and setting them to the side.
2. Heat your water in a pot, adding in your seaweed when it starts to boil. Cook for five minutes over medium heat.
3. Add your miso paste to a bowl, adding some hot water. Make sure to whisk until smooth, and then add to the soup.
4. Add in your green onion and tofu, stirring thoroughly.
5. Do not cook your miso paste. Serve warm.

Olive & Artichoke Tart

Serves: 4

Ingredients:

- 2 Cans Artichoke Hearts
- 2 Tablespoons Cornstarch
- 1 ½ Tablespoons Basil
- 1 ½ Teaspoons Oregano
- 4 Tablespoons Nutritional Yeast
- 2 Cloves Garlic
- 1 Lemon, Juiced
- 1 Tablespoon Mustard
- 1 Can Cannellini Beans
- ¾ Cup Cashews, Soaked
- ½ Cup Kalamata Olives, Pitted
- 1 Cup Peas, Frozen
- 1 Pack Vegan Puff Pastry
- 1 Tablespoon Summer Savory
- Sea Salt & Black Pepper to Taste

Directions:

1. Add your beans, mustard, cashews, garlic, lemon juice, herbs, starch, nutritional yeast, sea salt and pepper together. Add in 2/3 cup water, and then blend in a blender until smooth.

2. Press your puff pastry into your baking form, and then spread half of the cashew bean mixture to the bottom. Layer your artichoke hearts on top, and then your peas

and then your olives. Pour the rest of your bean mixture
on top.

3. Bake for thirty to forty minutes at 400 degrees before
letting it cool for five to ten minutes.

4. Serve warm.

Miso Onigiri

Serves: 8

Ingredients:

- 2 Cups Short Grain Sushi Rice, Washed & Drained, & Cooked (1 parts Rice to 1.2 parts water to make sticky rice)
- 2 Tablespoons Dulse Flakes
- 1 Tablespoon Miso Paste
- ½ Teaspoon Sea Salt, Fine
- 1 Tablespoon White Sesame Seeds, Toasted
- 1 Sheet Roasted Nori, Cut Into 8 Strips

Directions:

1. Divide your rice into eight portions before letting it cool.
2. In a wide shallow bowl, mix your sesame seeds and dulse flakes. Set it to the side, and then cut your nori strips before placing them to the side as well.
3. Fill a bowl with warm water, which will help you to handle the rice.
4. Wet your hands, sprinkling a pinch of salt onto your hands before you grab a portion of the rice. Make a loose ball before flattening it, and then use an indent with your finger before adding your filling. Add ½ teaspoon of miso paste into the center, forming your rice around it. Rotate and shape to get the desired shape, and then press two sides of your triangle into your toasted sesame seeds

and dulse flakes. Press the remaining side into the middle of the strip of nori. Fold the nori up on either side.

5. Repeat until you've made all of your onigiri.

Curried Lentils

Serves: 6

Ingredients:

- 1 Can Tomato Paste
- 2 Shallots
- 1 Jalapeno
- 4 Slices Ginger, Peeled
- 2 Cloves Garlic, Minced
- 2 Teaspoons Cumin
- 2 Teaspoon Ground Coriander
- 2 Cups Vegetable Broth
- 1 Can Coconut Milk, Light
- 1 ½ Cup Lentils
- 3 Cups Cauliflower Florets, Large
- 1 Cup Peas, Frozen
- 1/3 Cup Pistachios, Shelled, Chopped & Unsalted
- Basmati Rice, Cooked
- 1 Tablespoon Lime Juice, Fresh
- Sea Salt & Black Pepper to Taste

Directions:

1. Pulse your shallots, jalapeno, ginger, tomato paste, garlic, cumin, coriander, and a ½ teaspoon of salt and black pepper together. Transfer to a slow cooker bowl.

2. Add your lentils, broth, coconut milk and a cup of water. Stir until combined, and then put your cauliflower florets on top.

3. Cook on high for five hours.

4. Stir in lime juice, peas, and a dash more salt.

5. Serve with rice and garnished with pistachios.

Pumpkin Penne

Serves: 4

Ingredients:

- ½ Cup Unsalted Cashews, Soaked for 3-4 Hours, Drained & Rinsed
- 2 Tablespoon Olive Oil
- 16 Ounces Penne Pasta, Uncooked
- Sea Salt & Black Pepper to Taste
- ¾ Cup Vegetable Broth
- 5 Sage Leaves, Fresh
- Olive Oil for Drizzling
- 2 Garlic Cloves, Unpeeled & Minced
- ½ Yellow Onion, Sliced
- ½ Small Sugar Pumpkin, Diced

Directions:

1. Start by preheating your oven to 350. Line a baking sheet with foil, and then place your garlic, pumpkin and onion on it. Drizzle with olive oil, and then season with salt and pepper. Turn the pumpkin so the cut side is down, and then pierce it with a fork. Cover and bake for thirty-five to forty-five minutes.

2. Add your sage for the last five minutes. Remove the pan from heat, but keep it covered. Allow it to steam for another ten to fifteen minutes.

3. Pour your vegetable broth in a blender, and then remove the skin from the pumpkin. Add the pumpkin flesh to the

blender, blending. Add in your onion, peeled garlic, sage, cashews, sea salt and black pepper. Blend until smooth.

4. Prepare your pasta like you normally would, and then drain it.

5. Stir in your sauce, and serve while warm.

Quinoa & Mushroom Burgers

Serves: 4

Ingredients:

- 2 Tablespoons Canola Oil
- ¼ Cup Red Onion, Chopped
- ½ Cup Walnuts
- 4 Portobello Mushrooms Caps, Gills Removed & Chopped
- 3 Green Onions, Chopped
- 2 Teaspoon Rice Wine Vinegar
- 1 Cup Quinoa, Cooked
- Whole Grain Burger Buns
- ½ Cup Cornstarch
- Lettuce to Garnish
- Sliced Tomatoes to Garnish

Rosemary Mayonnaise:

- 1 Teaspoon Rosemary, Fresh & Chopped
- 1 Teaspoon Lemon Juice, Fresh
- ½ Cup Vegan Mayonnaise
- Sea Salt to Taste

Directions:

1. Start by making your burgers. You'll need to preheat the oven to 375, and then take a three quart shallow baking dish. Add your walnuts, garlic, mushrooms, a tablespoon oil, sea salt and pepper. Blake for twenty minutes. Your

mushroom should become tender, and then allow it to cool. Turn the oven off.

2. Pulse your mushroom mixture, green onions, red onions, and vinegar together in a food processor. Scrape the sides of the bowl if you need to, and transfer the mixture to a bowl, and then add in your cornstarch and quinoa. Stir until combined. Refrigerate while covered for two hours.

3. Preheat your oven to 375 again, and then prepare the baking sheet. From four to five patty mixtures.

4. Heat a tablespoon of oil over medium heat in a nonstick skillet, cooking your patties in batches. They should be browned, and they'll need flipped once during cooking.

5. Place your patties on the baking sheet, baking for ten minutes.

6. While your patties bake, add all of your rosemary mayonnaise ingredients together.

7. Assemble your burgers, topping with your lettuce and tomatoes before adding your rosemary mayonnaise to serve.

Buddha Bowl

Serves: 4

Ingredients:

- 1 Tablespoon Lemon Juice, Fresh
- 1 Small Clove Garlic, Minced
- 1 Avocado, Ripe & Diced
- ¼ Cup Cilantro, Chopped & Fresh
- 2 Cups Quinoa, Cooked
- 2 Tablespoon Water
- ½ Teaspoon Black Pepper, Divided
- 2 Tablespoons Tahini
- Sea Salt to Taste
- 3 Tablespoons Olive Oil, Divided
- 1 Sweet Potato, Cut into 1 Inch Chunks
- 15 Ounces Chickpeas, Rinsed

Directions:

1. Start by heating your oven to 425.
2. Toss your sweet potato in oil, and then add your salt and pepper. Transfer to a baking sheet, and then roast until tender for fifteen to eighteen minutes. You'll want to stir once in between.
3. Whisk your remaining oil with your water, tahini, and garlic and lemon juice. Add your sea salt and pepper, and then mix again.

4. Divide your quinoa into four bowls, and then add your toppings. Drizzle with tahini sauce and sprinkle with parsley before serving.

Dinner Recipes

Dinner can be hard to figure out and plan for, especially if you're trying to eat healthy. Luckily, with the vegan diet eating healthy can become a breeze. These dinner recipes are full of nutritional value, and you'll find that that many are quick to make too!

Lemon & Fettuccini "Alfredo"

Serves: 4

Ingredients:

- 4 Ounces Soy Cream Cheese
- 2 Cups Almond Milk, Unsweetened
- 12 Ounces Eggless Fettuccine
- 3 Tablespoons Nutritional Yeast + More for Garnish
- 1 Teaspoon Lemon Zest, Grated Fine
- ½ Cup Parsley, Chopped & Loosely Packed
- 3 Cloves Garlic, Chopped Fine
- 2 Tablespoons Olive Oil
- Sea Sal t& Black Pepper to Taste
- 3 Tablespoons Almonds, Blanked & Sliced

Directions:

1. Bring a pot of water to boil, cooking your noodles as per package instructions. Strain, and then reserve a cup of cooking water.

2. Add your soy cream cheese, almonds, almond milk, nutritional yeast, sea salt, pepper, and lemon zest together in a blender. Blend until smooth.

3. Heat your garlic and oil together over medium heat, stirring until the garlic starts to sizzle and soften. This should take one minute. Add in your soy milk mix, and then simmer until it's thick and creamy. You'll need to add ½ cup of your pasta water. It should take about eight minutes to cook.

4. Add in your fettuccini and parsley. Thin out as needed with more water.

5. Divide between bowl, and sprinkle with nutritional yeast before serving.

Soba Noodles & Ginger Sesame Sauce

Serves: 6

Ingredients:

Soba:

- 10 Ounces Sugar Snap Peas
- 6 Carrots, Peeled
- 2 Cups Edamame, Frozen
- 6 Ounces Soba Noodles
- ¼ cup Sesame Seeds
- ½ Cup Cilantro, Fresh & Chopped

Ginger Sesame Sauce:

- 1 Tablespoon Honey, Raw
- 1 Tablespoon White Miso (Vegan)
- 1 Teaspoon Chili Garlic Sauce
- 2 Teaspoon Ginger, Freshly Grated
- 1 Small Lime, Juiced
- 1 Tablespoon Toasted Sesame Oil
- 2 Tablespoons Peanut Oil
- ¼ Cup Tamari, Reduced Sodium

Directions:

1. Start by slicing your peas in half lengthwise. Slice your carrots into thin strips next.
2. Whisk together all sauce ingredients in a bowl until combined. Set this bowl to the side.
3. Bring two pots of water to a boil.

4. Toast your sesame seeds in a small pan for about four to five minutes over medium-low heat. Shake the pan to prevent burning. You'll need to shake or stir frequently. They should turn a golden brown, and you should be able to hear a soft popping noise.

5. In one pot, cook your soba noodles when it reaches a boil. Cook per package instructions before draining and rinsing under cool water briefly.

6. In your second pot, ad in your frozen edamame, cooking until warmed all the way through. This should take about four to six minutes, and then you can drain the.

7. Toss your peas into the boiling water, cooking for twenty seconds, and then drain your peas.

8. Combine your soba noodles, snap peas, edamame, and carrots. Pour in your dressing, and then toss.

9. Top with sesame seeds and cilantro before serving.

Coconut Curry

Serves: 4

Ingredients:

- 1 Tablespoon Coconut Oil
- 1 Small Onion, Diced
- 4 Cloves Garlic, Minced
- ½ Cup broccoli Florets, Diced
- 1 Tablespoon Ginger, Fresh & Grated
- ½ Cup Carrots, Diced
- ¼ Cup Tomatoes, Diced
- 1/3 Cup Snow Peas, Loosely Cut
- 1 Tablespoon Curry Powder
- 28 Ounces Light Coconut Milk, Canned
- 1 Cup Vegetable Stock
- Sea Salt & Black Pepper to Taste

Coconut Quinoa:

- 1 Tablespoon Agave Nectar
- 14 Ounces Light Coconut Milk, Canned
- 1 Cup Quinoa, Rinsed

For Garnish:

- Fresh Lemon Juice
- Cilantro, Chopped
- Red Pepper Flakes

Directions:

1. Wash your quinoa with a fine mesh strainer, and then add it to a saucepan. Turn the heat to medium, toasting it for three minutes. Add your can of light coconut milk and a half a cup of water before bringing it to a boil.

2. Reduce the heat, allowing it to simmer while covered for fifteen minutes. Your quinoa should be fluffy and all of the liquid should be absorbed. Set it to the side.

3. Heat a large saucepan using medium heat with a tablespoon of coconut oil in the pan. Once your oil is hot, add in your ginger, garlic, carrot, onion, broccoli, salt and pepper. Stir, and cook while stirring frequently for about five minutes.

4. Add in your curry powder, vegetable stock, and coconut milk. Add in a pinch of salt, and stir again. Bring it to a simmer before reducing the heat slightly, continuing to cook for ten to fifteen minutes.

5. Add in your snow peas and tomatoes, cooking for another five minutes. Be careful not to overcook your tomatoes.

6. Adjust the seasonings per your tastes, and then serve over your coconut quinoa.

Portobello Fajitas

Serves: 2

Ingredients:

- Sea Salt to Taste
- ½ Teaspoon Garlic Powder
- ½ Teaspoon Cumin
- 1 Teaspoon Steak Sauce
- 6 Small Corn Tortillas
- 2 Bell Peppers, Sliced Thin & Seeded
- 1 Tablespoon Coconut Oil
- 1 Poblano Pepper, Seeded & Sliced Thin
- 1 Jalapeno, Seeded & Sliced Thin
- 1 Yellow Onion, Cut Into Thin Rounds
- 2 Large Portobello Mushrooms, Steps Removed & Wiped Clean, Sliced Thin
- 2 Avocados, Ripe
- ½ Lime, Juiced
- Fresh Red Onion to Garnish
- Hot Sauce to Garnish
- Cilantro to Garnish
- Salsa to Garnish

Directions:

1. Eat a skillet over medium-high heat. Add in your oil, and then add in your pepper sand onions. Season with your salt, cumin and garlic.

2. Cook until your onions are softened and caramelized lightly. Make sure to stir often, and then set it aside. Keep it covered to keep them warm.

3. Add a dash of oil to the pan, and then add your mushrooms. Season with your salt, and once they're brown and softened add your vegan friendly steak sauce. Remove from heat, setting them to the side. Leave them covered to stay warm.

4. Add your avocados, lime juice, and seas salt to a bowl, mashing together. Mix well, and then add in your onion and cilantro.

5. Warm your tortillas in the oven or microwave, and then serve with pepper, onions, mushrooms, your homemade guacamole, and toppings.

Chili Mac & "Cheese"

Serves: 4

Ingredients:

- 1 Cup Raw Cashews, Soaked for 4-6 Hours & Drained
- 3-4 Cloves Garlic, Minced
- ½ White Onion, Diced
- 10 Ounces Macaroni Shells
- 1 ½ Cups Vegetable Broth
- 1 Tablespoon Cornstarch
- ½ Teaspoon Cumin
- 2 Tablespoons Nutritional Yeast
- ¾ Teaspoon Chili Powder
- 4 Ounces Diced Chilies, Canned

Directions:

1. Cook your pasta per package instructions.
2. Place a medium skillet over medium-low heat, sautéing your garlic and onion in your olive oil. Season with salt and pepper, stirring often. Continue to cook until fragrant and soft, which should take about seven minutes. Set this to the side.
3. Add your garlic and onion to a blender along with your remaining ingredients. Keep out half of your green chilies, blending until smooth.
4. Drain the noodles, setting them the side.
5. Place the cashew cheese in a pan, and cook until it thickens slightly.

6. Add in your macaroni noodles, stirring until combined.
    Add in your remaining green chilies, stirring again before
    serving.

Mushroom Stroganoff

Serves: 4

Ingredients:

- 1 Yellow Onion, Chopped
- 8 Ounces Ribbon Noodles, Uncooked
- 1 Tablespoon Olive Oil
- 3 Tablespoons White Wheat Flour, Divided
- 2 Cups Vegetable Broth
- 1 Tablespoon Soy Sauce
- 1 Teaspoon Tomato Paste
- 1 Teaspoon Lemon Juice
- 1 ½ lbs Mushrooms, Cut into 2 Inch Chunks
- ½ Teaspoon Thyme, Dried
- ½ Teaspoon Sage, Dried
- ½ Teaspoon Sea Salt, Fine
- 1 Tablespoon White Wine Vinegar
- Dah Black Pepper to Taste
- ¼ Cup Vegan Sour Cream (Optional)
- ¼ Cup Flat Leaf Parsley, Minced

Directions

1. Cook your noodles per package instructions, but under cook them just slightly. They will cook more when you place them in your sauce.

2. Drain your noodles and set them to the side. Add your olive oil, and sauté your onion for three minutes using medium heat.

3. Add your flour, cooking while stirring constantly for thirty seconds.

4. Add in your soy sauce, broth, lemon juice, and tomato paste gradually. Make sure that you keep stirring, and cook until it becomes thick and bubbly. This should take about a minute.

5. Add in your thyme, sage, salt and mushrooms, stirring to combine.

6. Cook for another five minutes while stirring frequently. Your mushrooms should shrink.

7. Add in your vinegar, simmering for another four minutes.

8. Add in your sour cream if you're using it. Add in your noodles, tablespoon of flour, pepper, and parsley, cooking for another five minutes on low. Remember to stir frequently.

9. Garnish with parsley before serving.

Mushroom Pho

Serves: 4

Ingredients:

- 64 Ounces Vegetable Broth, Low Sodium
- 6 Green Onions, Sliced Thin
- 1 Tablespoon Ginger, Fresh, Peeled & Grated
- Sea Salt to taste
- 1 ½ Tablespoons Vegan Butter Substitute
- 6 Ounces Shitake Mushrooms, Stems Removed
- 1 ½ Tablespoons Hoisin Sauce
- 2 Teaspoons Sesame Oil
- 14 Ounces Rice Noodles, Cooked
- 8 Ounces Bean Sprouts
- 2 Jalapeno Peppers, Sliced Thin
- Fresh Cilantro for Garnish

Directions:

1. Combine your vegetable broth, ginger, green onion and salt together in a large pot. Bring it to a boil, and then reduce the heat, letting it simmer for fifteen minutes.

2. Melt your butter substitute in a skillet using medium heat, and then add in your mushrooms. Sauté for six minutes. They should become tender, but you'll need to stir frequently to avoid burning.

3. Stir in your sesame oil and hoisin, cooking until your sauce thickens and coasts your mushrooms. Cook for about a minute more, and then remove it from heat.

4. Divide your rice noodles between four bowls, and then divide your ginger broth.

5. Add in your jalapeno, shiitake mushrooms, and cilantro. Drizzle with hoisin and chili garlic sauce before serving.

Garlic Pasta with Roasted Tomatoes

Serves: 4

Ingredients:

- 3 Cups Grape Tomatoes, Halved
- Olive Oil
- 10 Ounces Whole Wheat Pasta
- 8 Cloves Garlic, minced
- 2 Shallots, Diced
- Sea Salt & Black Pepper to Taste
- 4 Tablespoons All Purpose Flour
- 2 ½ Cups Almond Milk, Unsweetened

Directions:

1. Start by turning your oven to 400, and then toss your tomatoes in sea salt and olive oil.

2. Line a baking sheet with parchment paper, and then bake for twenty minutes. Set them aside once they're done.

3. Bring a large pot of water to boil, cooking your pasta as per package instructions. Drain and cover, and set them to the side.

4. In a large skillet, add a tablespoon of oil over medium-low heat. Add in your shallot and garlic, seasoning with salt and pepper. Cook for three to four minutes while stirring frequently. They should become softened and fragrant.

5. Stir in three to four tablespoons of flour, whisking constantly. Whisk in your almond milk, being careful so that it doesn't form clumps. Add another pinch of salt and black pepper, allowing to simmer for four to five minutes or until thickened.

6. Toss your pasta in your sauce, and top with roasted tomatoes before stirring.

7. Serve warm and garnished with fresh basil.

Curried Eggplant

Serves: 4

Ingredients:

- 1 Cup Basmati Rice
- 1 Tablespoon Olive Oil
- Sea Salt & Black Pepper to Taste
- 1 Onion, Chopped
- 2 Pints Cherry Tomatoes, Halved
- 1 Egg Plant, Cut into ½ Inch Pieces
- 1 ½ Teaspoons Curry Powder
- 15.5 Ounces Chickpeas, Canned & Rinsed
- ½ Cup Basil, Fresh
- ¼ Cup Low Fat Vegan Yogurt, Optional

Directions:

1. In a medium saucepan, combine your rice, 1 ½ cups water, and a half teaspoon of sea salt. Bring it to a boil, stir once, and then cover. Reduce the heat to low, allowing it to simmer for eighteen minutes. Remove from heat, allowing it to sit while covered for five more minutes.

2. Heat your oil over medium-high heat in a medium skillet. Add in your onion, cooking while stirring occasionally. Cook until softened which should take four to six minutes.

3. Add in your eggplant, curry powder, sea salt, black pepper and tomatoes. Stir and cook until fragrant. This should take about two minutes.

4. Add in two cups of water, bringing it to a boil. Reduce the heat, allowing it to simmer partially covered for twelve to fifteen minutes. Your eggplant should become tender.

5. Stir in your chickpeas, cooking until they're heated all the way through. This should take about three more minutes.

6. Remove from heat and stir in basils.

7. Serve over rice, and garnished with vegan yogurt.

Spicy Coconut Noodles

Serves: 4

Ingredients:

- 13.5 Ounces Coconut Milk, Canned & Unsweetened
- 8 Ounces Rice Noodles
- 3 Tablespoons Tomato Paste
- 1 Teaspoon Chili Powder
- 1 Teaspoon Sea Salt, Fine
- 1 Tablespoon Chili Paste
- 3 Scallions, Sliced Thin
- 8 Ounces Bean Sprouts
- 16 Basil Leaves, Torn & Fresh
- ¼ Cup Coconut, Shredded & Toasted

Directions:

1. Cook your noodles per package instructions. Drain and set them to the side.
2. Take a large saucepan and place it over medium-high heat. Combine your tomato paste, coco nut milk, salt, chili paste and chili powder.
3. Bring it to a boil, and then reduce to a simmer. Allow it to simmer for two to three minutes.
4. Stir in your drained noodles, and then toss.
5. Divide between bowls, topping with your toasted coconut before serving.

Dessert Recipes

Here are some vegan desert recipes that everyone is sure to enjoy! Just because you choose the vegan diet doesn't mean you have to go without your sweet desserts.

Cashew & Coconut Rice Pudding

Serves: 4

Ingredients:

- 1 Cup Coconut Milk, Unsweetened
- 1 Teaspoon Vanilla Extract, Pure
- 3 Tablespoons Raw Sugar
- ¼ Cup Arborio Rice
- ½ Cup Cashews, Raw
- 2 Teaspoons Lime Zest, Finely Grated
- Fresh Berries to garnish

Directions:

1. Start by placing your cashews in a blender with a cup of water. Puree until smooth.
2. Add your coconut milk, rice, cashew milk, sugar, and lime zest in a saucepot, whisking until smooth and bringing it to a simmer using medium heat.
3. Cover loosely, allowing it to simmer gently while stirring often for about twenty-five minutes. Your rice should become tender.

4. Remove from heat, stirring in your vanilla.

5. Allow it to cool before chilling.

6. Serve garnished with fresh berries.

Blueberry Muffins

Serves: 12

Ingredients:

- 2 Cups Blueberries

- ½ Cup Vegetable Oil

- ½ Cup Soy Milk

- ¼ Cup Agave Nectar

- ½ Cup Maple Syrup, Pure

- ½ Teaspoon Sea Salt, Fine

- 2 Teaspoons Baking Powder

- 2 Cups Whole Wheat Spelt Flour

Directions:

1. Start by preheating your oven to 375, and then line a mini cupcake tin with paper cups.

2. Mix all of your dry ingredients together in one bowl.

3. Mix all of your wet ingredients together in a separate bowl.

4. Combine your dry and wet ingredients, and then fold in your blueberries.

5. Divide the batter between your muffin tins, filling them almost to the top.

6. Bake until golden brown, which should take about twenty
    minutes.

Double Chocolate Cookies

Yields: 12-20

Ingredients:

- 2 ¼ Cups Whole Wheat Flour
- 1 Teaspoon Baking Soda
- ½ Cup Dutch Processed Cocoa, Unsweetened
- 1 Cup Vegan Butter Substitute
- 1 ¼ Cup Sugar
- ½ Teaspoon Sea Salt
- 2 Teaspoons Vanilla Extract, Pure
- 1 Tablespoon Molasses, Unsulfured
- ¼ Cup Almond Milk
- 1 Cup Vegan Chocolate Chips

Directions:

1. Start by heating your oven to 350.
2. Sift your cocoa, salt, baking soda and flour together before setting it to the side.
3. In a separate bowl you'll need to ream your vanilla, sugar, butter substitute and molasses together until creamy. It should become fluffy.
4. Add in your almond milk, mixing well.
5. Mix your wet ingredients into your dry ingredients, stirring to combine.
6. Add in your chocolate chips.

7. Scoop ¼ cup of the cookie dough, rolling it into a ball. Flatten slightly, and then repeat until you've used up all of your dough.
8. Bake for ten minutes.
9. Cook while on a baking sheet for five minutes.
10. Transfer to a cooking rack, letting stand for ten to fifteen minutes before serving.

Chocolate Cupcakes

Yields: 15

Ingredients:

Cupcakes:

- ½ Teaspoon Baking Soda
- 1 Teaspoon Baking Powder
- 1 Cup Sugar
- 1 ½ Cups All Purpose Flour
- ¼ Cup Dutch Process Cocoa Powder
- ¼ Teaspoon Ground Cinnamon
- ¼ Tablespoon Sea Salt, Fine
- 1 Cup Almond Milk, Unsweetened
- 1 Tablespoon Balsamic Vinegar
- 1 Teaspoon Vanilla Extract

Frosting:

- ½ Cup Dutch Process Cocoa Powder, Sifted
- 1 Teaspoon Vanilla Extract, Pure
- 1/3 Cup Coconut Oil
- ¼ Cup Light Brown Sugar, Packed
- 2 Cups Icing Sugar, Sifted
- 6 Tablespoons Almond Milk

Directions:

1. Start by turning your oven to 350, and then line a muffin tin with fifteen paper liners. You may need two muffin tins.

2. Sift your sugar, cocoa, baking powder, flour, salt, baking soda and cinnamon into a large whisking bowl. Add in your oil, balsamic vinegar, almond milk and vanilla. Make sure to whisk well, and continue whisking until you get a smooth batter. Spoon into your paper cups.

3. Bake for about twenty minutes. A toothpick should be able to be inserted into the middle and come out clean.

4. Allow to cool while you make your frosting. Your cupcakes need to be completely cooled before you add your frosting.

5. Beat your coconut oil and brown sugar together until smooth, and then add in your cocoa powder and vanilla. Beat well.

6. Stir in a cup of icing sugar, beating until smooth and then add in your almond milk. Continue to bet, and then add in your remaining icing sugar. Continue to beat until smooth and fluffy.

7. Spread over your cupcakes, and chill before serving.

Set Strawberries & Coconut Cream

Serves: 4

Ingredients:

- 13.5 Ounces Coconut Milk, Canned
- 2 Tablespoons chia Seeds
- 2 Cup Strawberries, Fresh & Stalks Removed
- 1 Teaspoon Vanilla Extract, Pure
- 1 Teaspoon Maple Syrup, Pure
- 4 Fresh Strawberries to Garnish
- Fresh Mint Leaves to Garnish
- Lemon Zest to Garnish

Directions:

1. Chill your coconut milk.
2. Blend your strawberries in a food processor until smooth, adding in your chia seeds. Stir, and then divide between four ramekins. Refrigerate for an hour or overnight.
3. Open your coconut milk, scooping the creamy top part and leave the liquid separated.
4. Add your vanilla, cinnamon and maple syrup with your coconut cream. Whip until fluffy. You need to be careful to not over whip.
5. Spoon the cream into each ramekin.
6. Garnish with mint, strawberries and lemon zest to serve.

Chocolate Pie

Serves: 8

Ingredients:

- 12.3 Ounces Extra Firm, Silken Tofu
- 1 ½ Teaspoons Vanilla Extract, Pure
- 3 Tablespoons Almond Milk
- Sea Salt to Taste
- 2 Tablespoons Maple Syrup, Pure
- 1 ½ Cups Vegan Dark Chocolate Chips

Crust:

- 2 Tablespoons Brown Sugar
- 12 Graham Cracker Sheets
- ¼ Cup Coconut Oil, Melted

Directions:

1. You'll want to start by making your curst. Turn your oven to 375. Place your sugar and crackers in the food processor. Pulse until they're combined. Drizzle in your coconut oil, pulsing a few more times. The crust should start to hold together.
2. Press your crust into a pie pan, baking for eight to ten minutes. It should become golden brown, and you'll need to give your crust time to cool.
3. Add your vanilla, almond milk, sea salt, tofu, and maple syrup to the food processor or blender, blending well. Melt your chips using a double boiler, adding them into the tofu mixture. Blend again.

4. Pour the filling into your crust, letting it set in the fridge for a minimum of three hours before slicing and serving chilled.

Snickerdoodles

Serves: 18

Ingredients:

- 1 Cup Sugar
- ½ Cup Butter Substitute
- 1 ½ Cups Flour
- ¼ Teaspoon Cream of Tartar
- ¼ Teaspoon Baking Powder
- 1 Prepared Egg Replacement
- 1 Teaspoon Vanilla Extract, Pure
- Cinnamon for Rolling

Directions:

1. Cream your butter replacement, vanilla and sugar together. Add your egg replacement, whipping until it's fluffy.
2. Whisk all of your dry ingredients besides your cinnamon together.
3. Add 2/3 of the dry ingredients to your whipped mixture. Whip to combine. Add in your remaining flour, making sure to mix by hand.
4. Cover the dough using plastic wrap, refrigerating for an hour.
5. Heat your oven to 375. Once your dough is chilled, prepare a cookie sheet with parchment paper.
6. Use an ice cream scoop to make balls from your dough, and then roll the balls in cinnamon.

7. Squish them down with a fork, and then cook for ten to twelve minutes. Ten minutes will produce chewy cookies and twelve minutes will produce crunch cookies.
8. Let them cool for thirty seconds before removing them from the baking sheet.

Plum Kuchen

Serves: 8

Ingredients:

- 1 ½ Teaspoon Lemon Zest, Fresh
- 2 Teaspoon Egg Replacement
- ½ Teaspoon Sea Salt
- 1 Cup Sugar, Divided
- 2 Cups All Purpose Flour + 2 Tablespoons, Divided
- ¼ Cup Warm Water
- 2 ¼ Teaspoon Active Dry Yeast
- 1 Teaspoon Vanilla Extract, Pure
- ½ Cup + 2 Tablespoons Vegan Butter Replacement, Divided
- ¾ lbs Ripe Plums, Halved & Pitted
- ½ Cup + 1 Tablespoon Tofutti Sour Cream (or Vegan Yogurt)

Directions:

1. Combine your yeast and water together before setting it aside until it become slightly foamy.
2. In a bowl combine your yeast, two cups of flour, 2/3 cup sugar, sour cream, egg substitute, vanilla extract and lemon zest.
3. Beat on low until all ingredients are combined, and then mix for five minutes. Add in ½ cup of your vegan butter one tablespoon at a time while mixing.

4. Beat for five more minutes on medium speed. It should become sticky, smooth and shiny.

5. Remove your bowl from the mixer, and then top with the remaining 2 tablespoons of flour. Don't overmix it, and then cover with a kitchen towel. Set it aside for ninety minutes to two hours.

6. Mix your dough after the first rise, combining the flour that's on top.

7. Grease your 9x9 cake pan with the remaining two tablespoons of vegan butter. Sprinkle the remaining 1/3 cup of sugar onto the bottom of your pan.

8. Halve and pit your plums. Slice your pitted plums if they're large. Place them over the bottom of the pan.

9. Pour the dough over the plumps, letting it rise for another ninety minutes. Cover with oiled plastic wrap.

10. Heat your oven to 375, and bake for thirty-five minutes. It should become golden and slightly cracked.

11. Take it out of the oven, letting it rest for five m minutes before loosening the oven.

12. Turn it over onto the rack to cool before cutting to serve.

Easy Brownies

Serves: 8

Ingredients:

- ¾ Cup All Purpose Flour
- ¾ Teaspoon Baking Powder
- ¼ Teaspoon Sea Salt, Fine
- ½ Cup Dutch Process Cocoa Powder
- 1 Teaspoon Vanilla Extract, Pure
- 2 Large Flax Eggs
- ¾ Cup Cane Sugar
- ½ Cup Non-Dairy Butter
- 1/3 Cup Walnuts, Chopped

Directions:

1. Start by preheating your oven to 350, and then spray a seven to eight standard muffin tins or use paper liners.
2. Prepare your flax eggs letting them rest in a bowl for five minutes.
3. Put your butter in a microwave safe bowl, melting it. Add in your sugar, vanilla, baking powder, flax eggs, cocoa powder and salt. Whisk well.
4. Add in your flour, mixing well before folding in your walnuts.
5. Scoop your batter into your muffin tins, and then bake for twenty-two to twenty-six minutes. The brownies should start to pull away from the sides.
6. Allow to cool before serving.

Conclusion

Now you have all the recipes you need to get started on your vegan diet! The vegan diet is an easy way to lose weight and meet all of your health goals. By cutting out meat and other animal products, you cut out a large amount of cholesterol and unhealthy fats, leaving you with lean and healthy ingredients to make healthy meals. With so many great recipes to choose from, there's no reason not to go vegan and still enjoy your day to day meals. Just find a recipe that sounds like it'll delight your taste buds, and try the vegan diet today!

www.ingramcontent.com/pod-product-compliance
Lightning Source LLC
Chambersburg PA
CBHW050648250726

48662CB00002B/554